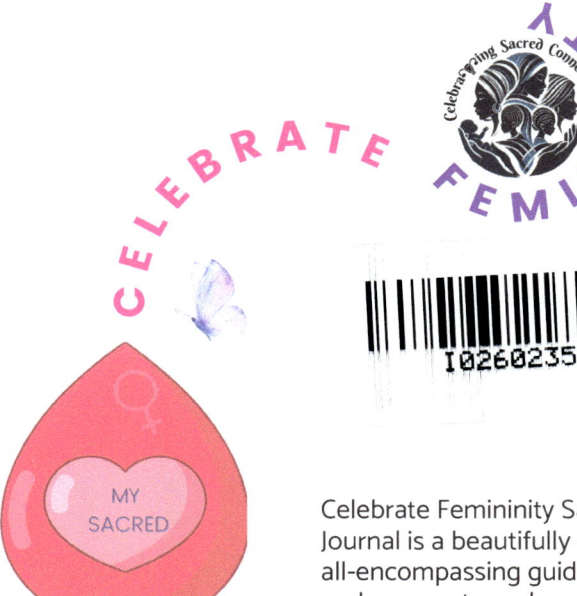

Celebrate Femininity Sacred Journal is a beautifully designed, all-encompassing guide for girls and women to embrace and honor their menstrual cycle.

Small enough to fit in most handbags, this journal is an educational tool and companion that provides thoughtful prompts for each phase of your cycle, helping you connect with your body and emotions. It includes planning pages to support holistic well-being through the womb foods one eats, joyful movement, self-reflection exercises, a monthly planner, and a menstrual tracker to keep you organized and mindful.

With space to celebrate your inner beauty, strength, and wisdom, this journal serves as a sacred tool for the empowered female to celebrate, take control, ensure self-care and deeper connection to the rhythm of your femininity.

Celebrating Sacred Connections

ISBN: 979-8-9896332-3-4

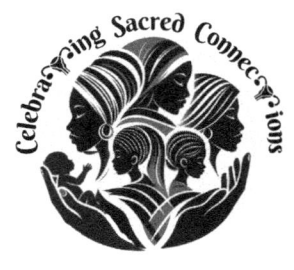

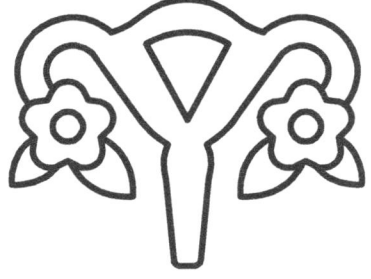

My Sacred Journal

Celebrating Sacred Connections

ISBN: 979-8-9896332-3-4
Published by Shakir Enterprises
in collaboration with Wombniverse Gallery
October 2024
Atlanta, Georgia
United States of America, USA

Copyrighted 2024
All rights reserved. No part of this book may be reproduced or used in any manner without the prior written permission of the copyright owner, except for the use of brief quotations in a book review.

celebratingsacredconnections@gmail.com

PREFACE

What comes to mind when you hear the words feminine, grace, womanhood, femininity, or anything associated with being a woman, girl, or female? Those very thoughts are the inspiration for this journal and our movement. We believe in the majesty and great honor of women (wombmen) --the wombs of all minds and beings.

Welcome to a journal that celebrates the Divine design of women, femininity, and the sacred power of the womb. This space has been created for you to explore, reflect, and embrace the fullness of your femininity—a force that is beautiful on the surface and profoundly powerful in its depths.

Throughout history, the essence of femininity has often been misunderstood or minimized, portrayed as weakness or vulnerability. Yet, in truth, being soft is a superpower. It is within softness that we find the capacity for immense strength, resilience, and grace. Like water, we flow with the currents of life, adapting, nourishing, and sustaining those around us while holding an inner power that is unshakable.

This journal is an invitation to reclaim the majesty of being a wombman. You are Divinely crafted by the Creator, and within you lies a sacred energy that is both creative and life-giving. Whether you are reflecting on the cycles of your body, the wisdom of your intuition, or the strength of your heart, let these pages serve as a sanctuary where you can reconnect with the liberty of your femininity.

Here, we honor the womb, a symbol of creation and transformation. Beyond the physical, we also celebrate the womb of ideas, dreams, and purpose that women carry. Your ability to nurture and birth new life, whether in the form of children, relationships, projects, change in the world we live in, or visions for the future, is a testament to your strength.

As you journal, remember that your beauty may be defined by what is seen on the surface—it is also in the way you love, create, heal, and grow. This journal is a place to redirect your energies, honor your softness, and stand tall in the glory of your wombmanhood. Through these reflections, may you discover and celebrate the liberty of being exactly who you are—a wombman of Divine design, whose strength and beauty radiate from the inside out. As you continue to grow into the evolved self, stand strong in our new reality.

celebratingsacredconnections@gmail.com

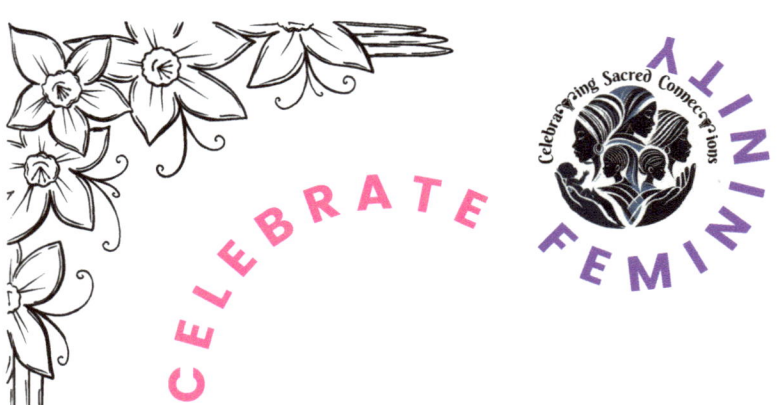

We are so grateful that you are present with Celebrating Sacred Connections and the Wombniverse Gallery as we celebrate femininity. We celebrate femininity by getting in touch with our inner beauty and establishing balance in our lives. We'd like to start by defining terms as they are used in this wonderful journal. You will see that our reference to the female is wombman. That is because it is celebratory to recognize and hold a torch for the fact that every human being who has ever lived on Earth has come through the womb of a wombman.

As we honor wombmen, we are also conscious of the contribution of the male/man. This is to be ever aware of balance in our lives. We define man as meaning mind and wombman is the womb of mind. The wombman has a womb and a mind.

Celebrate!!!   (See the glossary for further word exploration)

The term femininity is rich in meaning and balances the masculine attributes. Looking at the word femininity, we see "fem" meaning wombman. "Female" meaning wombman (environment for development of the mind).   In human beings, female is the gender which brings forth new life. She is most often the primary teacher and caretaker. The feminine (note the nine~at the end of fem, as in nine months of gestation), attributes that we share with you at this time are, to name a few: openness, softness, contemplative, nurturing, feeling, receiving, listening, intuition, poise, tranquility, gracefulness, composure, rest and knowing.

Adilah & Madame Q

celebratingsacredconnections@gmail.com

GLOSSARY
TERMS TO KNOW

The glossary in this publication is to expand understanding of the wombman and femininity as we drill deeper into the wonderful world of wombmanhood. It is the result of so many years of negativity and whispers around the beautiful menstrual cycle and the myriad gifts that come with it.

In many communities and groups, it is disdained. Oftentimes, young girls are not properly introduced to the wonders of wombmanhood and its responsibilities.

This glossary borrows from the school of Nunetics to share the meanings of consonant letters to help one think differently about terms one may have had contact with before, but now we introduce another way of looking at them. Enjoy!

B	THE ABDOMEN, THE TESTICLES, ANY CONTAINER WHICH EMPTIES AND REFILLS, IN, WITH
F	RELATED TO BODY PART: NOSE, NOSTRILS, LIPS. LIVING THINGS THAT CLEAVE OR BREATHE, DAYBREAK-BRINGING IN NEW AIR, SUSTAINS LIFE BY BREATHING, INTUITION, NATIVE INTELLIGENCE

L	THE TONGUE. TASTING, TALKING, KISSING. LANGUAGE. COMMUNICATION. DISCERNMENT. TO DRAW SEPARATIONS AND DISTINCTIONS BETWEEN THINGS
M	RELATED TO THE STOMACH, A CONTAINED AREA THAT SHRINKS AND GROWS CIRCUMSTANTIALLY, SUBSTANCE MADE MALLEABLE AND ENTERING THE STOMACH'S SEMI-FLUID ENVIRON, MULTIPLICITY OF ACCUMULATION, KNOWLEDGE AND UNDERSTANDING, MOTHERING, NURTURING.
N	LIFE GERM SEED, SPERMATOZOA, BREATH THROUGH EXHALATION, UPWARD MOVEMENT, EASING OF BURDENS, EASE, GENTLENESS, SIMPLICITY, AROMA, THINGS HINTED AT, SECRETS, RUMORS
R	FRONT OF HEAD. ROUNDNESS OF THE FACE WITH CIRCULAR ORIFICES-- EYEBALLS, EARS, OPEN MOUTH, NOSTRILS, TO MOVE FORWARD AT A RAPID PACE. REACH THE TOP. AUTHORITY. COMMAND. CONSCIOUSNESS.
T	HAIR-WHEN GROOMED, CUT OR PLUCKED, TIE, TETHER, TWO INDEPENDENT THINGS CONNECTED, RECIPROCAL RELATIONSHIPS, BENEATH THE SURFACE.
W	FACIAL CHEEKS, BUTTOCKS, CONNECTIONS DESIGNED TO ACCOMMODATE THE INCLUSION OR EXCLUSION OF A THING, THINGS UNIVERSAL
Y	OPEN, OUTSTRETCHED HAND, BRINGING IN AND GIVING OUT, HANDLE YOUR BUSINESS, YEAST, THE ENVIRONMENT, STRETCHING THE IMAGINATION

How to Make Great Use of This Journal

This Celebrate Femininity Sacred Journal is designed as a guide for women to connect deeply with their bodies, minds, and spirits throughout each phase of the menstrual cycle. This journal is a sacred space where you can document your experiences, track patterns, reflect on your thoughts and feelings, and celebrate the Divine design of your feminine self. By journaling through each phase of your cycle, you can gain insights that allow you to nurture yourself more fully and evolve each month.

1. Track Foods Eaten

Your diet plays a significant role in how you feel throughout your cycle. Use this journal to note the foods you consume and observe how they affect your energy, mood, and physical symptoms.

- During the Menstrual Phase: Reflect on how certain foods—like warming soups, iron-rich vegetables, or herbal teas—make you feel. Are you craving specific nutrients or comfort foods? How does your body respond?
- During the Follicular Phase: Notice how your energy begins to rise. Do lighter, fresher foods (like fruits, salads, or smoothies) feel more appealing? Track how eating habits evolve as your body prepares for ovulation.
- During the Ovulatory Phase: As you feel more energetic, do you notice a shift in your food preferences? Pay attention to how your body feels with different food choices.
- During the Luteal Phase: As your body prepares for menstruation, track how cravings for comfort foods or richer meals change. Do certain foods help ease symptoms like bloating, mood swings, or fatigue?

2. Record Activities and Movement

Your body's energy levels fluctuate throughout the month, and this journal is a way to align your physical activities with your cycle.

- Menstrual Phase: Note the level of physical activity your body feels comfortable with. Is your body asking for rest, gentle yoga, or meditation? Write down any activities that support relaxation and restoration.
- Follicular Phase: As your energy increases, document any activities that energize you, such as exercise, walking, or creative projects. How does physical movement help fuel your creativity or productivity during this time?

How to make Great use of *This Journal*

③ Capture Ideas and Inspirations

The phases of your cycle can spark different types of creativity, introspection, and mental clarity. Use this journal to capture ideas that arise during each phase.

- **Menstrual Phase:** This phase is a time of reflection and release. What ideas or realizations come to you when you allow yourself to rest? Journal any thoughts that surface as you tune into our inner wisdom. Record dreams.
- **Follicular Phase:** Creativity often flows easily during this phase. Write down any new ideas, goals, or projects that you're excited about. Reflect on how your mental clarity allows for new possibilities.
- **Ovulatory Phase:** During this time, you may feel more communicative, inspired, highly energetic, and increased social interests. Document any ideas for collaborations, social connections, or projects that come to mind.
- **Luteal Phase:** As your energy turns inward, you may notice insights or reflections that hel you prepare for the next cycle. Use this time to note any ideas related to sel care, personal growth, or completing tasks.

Inspiration

④ Reflect on Concerns and Emotio

Throughout each phase of your cycle, you may experience a range of emotions. Use this journal to process and reflect on your feelings.

- Menstrual Phase: What emotions are you releasi during this time? How can you honor them witho judgment? Journaling during this phase allows yo to let go of what no longer serves you.
- Follicular Phase: As your mood lifts, how do you feel emotionally? Write about the excitement or optimism that comes with this phase. What are y looking forward to, and how do you want to approach the weeks ahead?
- Ovulatory Phase: You may feel more open and connected. Reflect on how your emotional state influences your interactions with others. Are the any relationships or dynamics you're feeling particularly grateful for?
- Luteal Phase: Premenstrual emotions can be intense. Use the journal to explore any concerns anxieties that arise. Reflect on how your body is signaling the need for rest and nurturing.

How to make Great use of *This Journal*

 Answer the Journal Prompts

This journal includes guided questions to help you reflect more deeply on each phase of your cycle. Use the prompts to direct your thoughts and bring awareness to your experiences. You may also create your own questions as you become more attuned to your cycle.

Menstrual Phase: "What do I need to release this month, physically or emotionally?"

Follicular Phase: "What new intentions or goals am I setting for myself?"

- **Ovulatory Phase:** "How can I use my high energy to nurture my relationships or creative pursuits?"
- **Luteal Phase:** "What self-care practices can I focus on as I prepare for the next cycle?"

 **Reflect and Evolve Each Month**

At the end of each cycle, review your journal entries to notice patterns and insights. What did you learn about your body, your emotions, and your creativity? Use these reflections to evolve your self-care practices, your diet, and your approach to work and relationships for the next cycle.

This journal is a sacred tool to help you honor the rhythms of your body and the Divine power of your femininity. **Through each phase of your cycle,** you are reminded of the strength, beauty, and wisdom that lies within you.

Let this journal guide your journey toward deeper self-awareness, growth, and empowerment.

Menstrual Cycle Phases

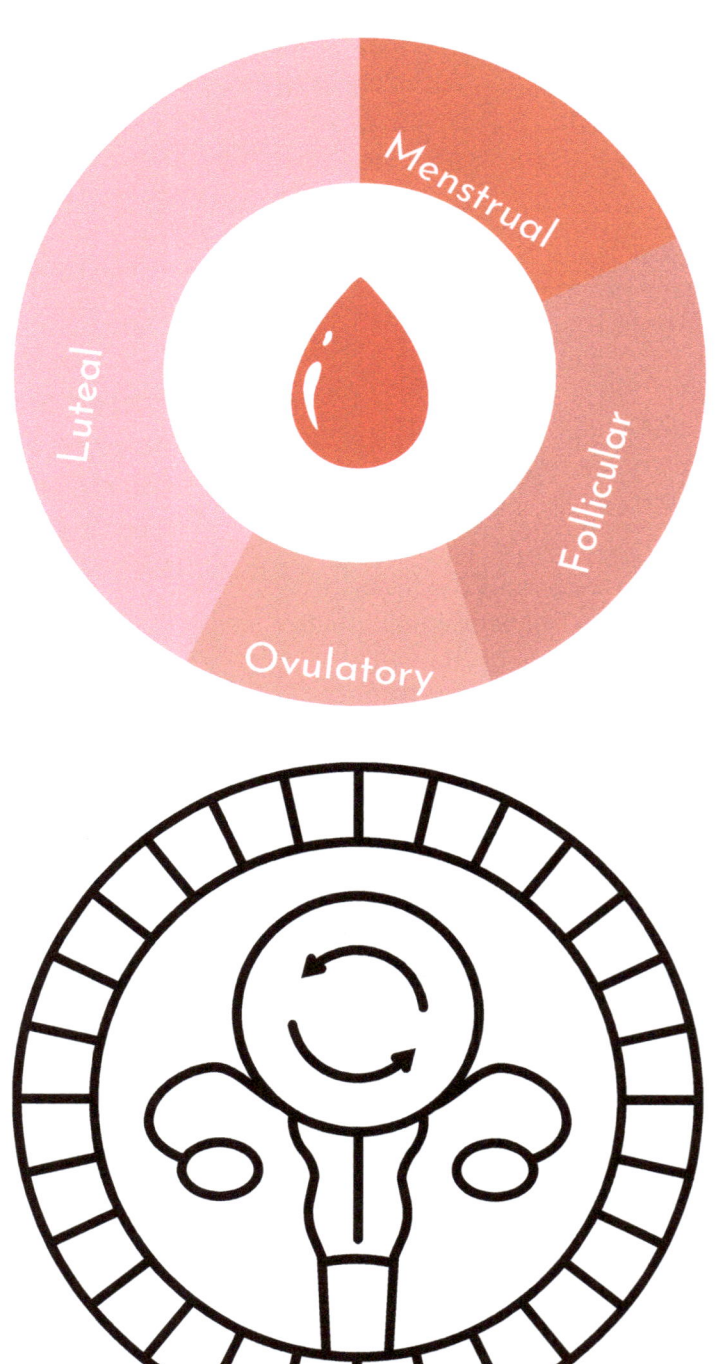

Benefits of a Writing Journal, Diary, or Keepsake Messages

Journaling is a practice of writing one's thoughts and feelings, recording memories or finding self-expression.

Relieve Stress

Surely, reflecting benefits the reflector.

The journal writing method of expressing one's self can be therapeutic as it may unleash valuable self-knowledge, solve problems, or help relieve any stress or uneasiness one may feel or think.

journal to have a personal, self-scussion, to get a r understanding of eriences and/or to ument one's growth, concerns, needs, ideas, or wants.

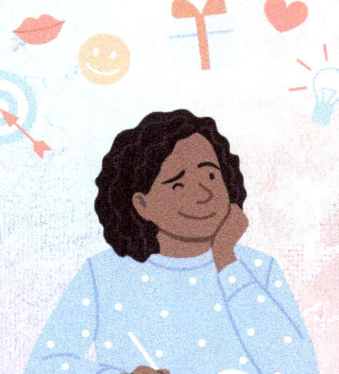

Keep your thoughts organized

Boost Your Mamory

Write as much as you want or need. It's your release, reflect, connect time just for you!!!

Record ideas on-the-go.

Enhance your writing skills

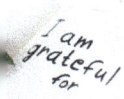
I am grateful for

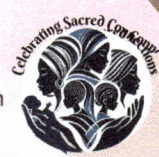

celebratingsacredconnections@gmail.com

Writing Journal

Surely, reflecting benefits the reflector

Reflect, think, write in your journal as often as you desire, especially during the time of your bleed days.

- How do I demonstrate that I regard my womb as precious?
- What are ways that I communicate, listen, and respond to my womb?
- How am I listening to hear the messages of my womb?
- During the time of menstruation, how do I take time to be still, observe and track the cycle, check for new bleeding color, clots, texture, (thick or thin), odor, changes day to day, period to period?
- Does my bleeding start bright red and end bright red?
- Is my cycle 28-30 days?

You can write about the following statements and questions:

- What is the state of my relationship with the Creator?
- What is the state of my relationship with my womb?
- How do I give thought, attention, care and love to womb?

- What do I feel days before, days after the period? Track and make notes each day of my cycle How does what's going on in my life affect my cycle?
- How will I make this wonderful time to slow down, spend time in introspection, take note be a time to be especially kind to myself?

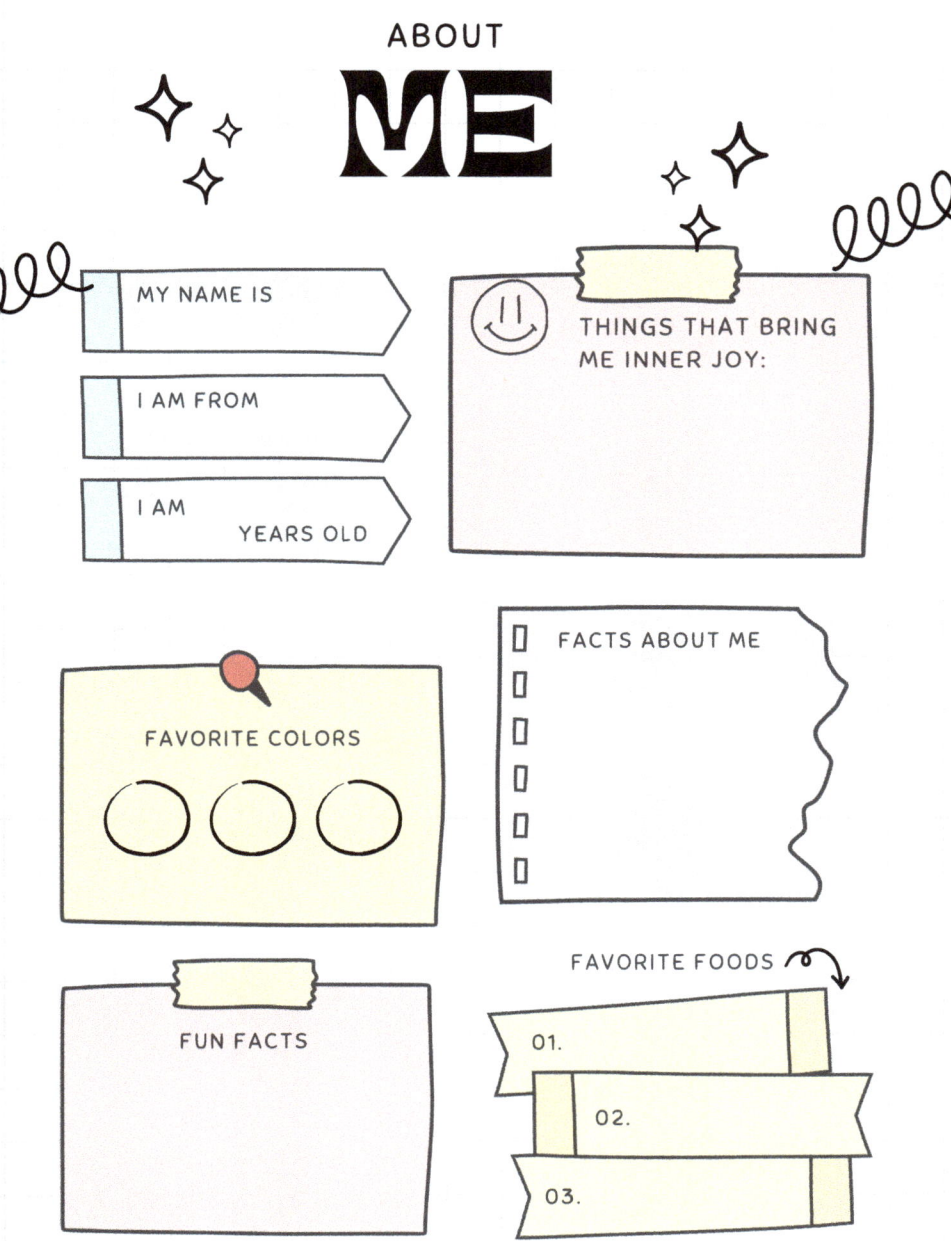

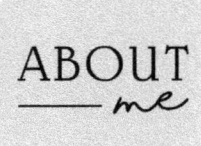

ABOUT me

REFLECTIONS
HOW DO YOU FEEL ABOUT WHO YOU ARE, THE THINGS THAT MAKE YOU WHO YOU ARE? WHAT MAKES YOU SO BEAUTIFUL?

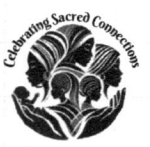

My Maternal Lineage

Honoring the Wombs that Bore Me
Me - My Name is

Knowing and acknowledging one's maternal lineage is important because it connects us to the wisdom, strength, and experiences of the women whose DNA we share, shaping our identity and grounding us in our heritage.

Knowing and acknowledging one's maternal lineage is a way to honor the legacy of resilience, love, and tradition passed down through generations, fostering a deeper understanding of ourselves and our place in the world

My Mother's Name:
Facts and Info about her:

My Grandmother's Name
Facts and Info about her:

My Great Grandmother's Name
Facts and Info about her:

My Great, Great Grandmother's Name
Facts and Info about her:

My Great, Great, Great Grandmother's Name
Facts and Info about her:

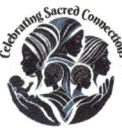

MY MATERNAL LINEAGE

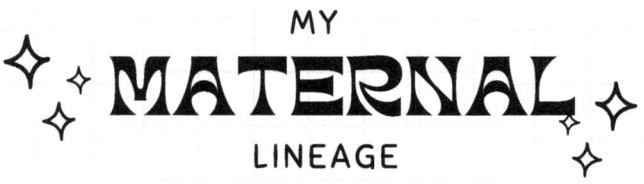

WHAT ARE COMMON TRENDS, CHARACTER TRAITS, AND ATTRIBUTES OF YOUR MATERNAL LINEAGE DO YOU SEE REPEATING ITSELF? WHAT HAVE YOU INHERITED FROM YOUR MATERNAL MOTHER AND GRANDMOTHERS? HOW DID THEY MOVE IN THE COMMUNITY? WITH WHAT DID THEY OCCUPY THEMSELVES? WHAT ABOUT THEIR HEALTH STATES?

(Hint: It may be more pronounced in some than others, but it is very prevalent and common to most of the women in your family.)

The Language of Body Talk

How is my body communicating with me today? What sensations am I noticing—such as tingles, pressure, softness, numbness, or other subtle feelings? How do these signals speak to my needs, emotions, or overall well-being?

Thank you!

FOR WHAT ARE YOU THANKFUL? WRITE ABOUT AS MANY THINGS AS YOU CAN TO EXPRESS GRATITUDE.

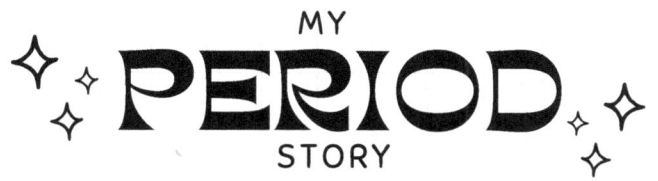

MY PERIOD STORY

WHEN DID YOU HAVE YOUR FIRST PERIOD? WERE YOU PREPARED FOR IT? WHO WAS WITH YOU? WHAT HAPPENED? WHAT WERE YOU FEELING? HOW WAS THAT FIRST PERIOD --THOSE BLEED DAYS?

PURPOSE OF THE FEMALE ORGANS

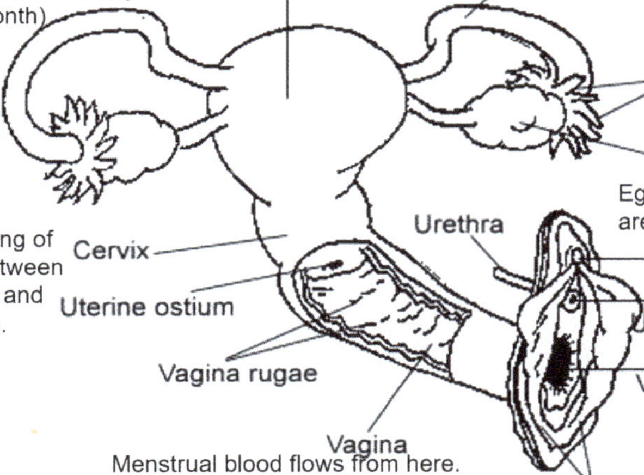

The egg cell passes along here once released from the ovary (once a month) — Uterine tube

Fetus grows and develops during pregnancy — Uterus

- Fimbriae
- **Ovary** — Egg cells called ova are produced here
- Urethra
- Clitoris
- Urethral opening
- Vaginal orifice
- Labia minora
- Labia majora (not pictured) - outer folds of skin that protect the female genitals

This is a ring of muscle between the uterus and the vagina. — Cervix

- Uterine ostium
- Vagina rugae

Vagina — Menstrual blood flows from here. This is where the sperm is deposited by the penis during sexual intercourse.

How does it feel to know the purpose of your female organs? What will you do with this knowledge?

ABOUT THE FEMININE DESIGN

FALLOPIAN TUBES
These are the thin, soft tubes extending from the uterus to the ovaries.

UTERUS
It is a hollow, pear-shaped organ with a muscular wall and a lining.

CERVIX
It is located in the lower portion of the uterus that opens into the vagina.

OVARIES
These are the female reproductive organs.

VAGINA
It is the outside passage way of the baby which is called as the "birth canal."

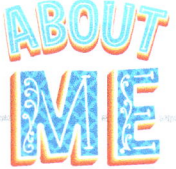 and my feminine design

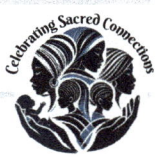

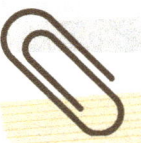

I am fueled by happy thoughts.

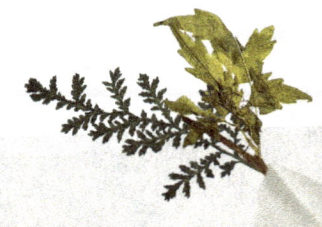

FUN FACTS

ABOUT THE MOON

& WORDS FROM "MOON"

MOON
heavenly body which revolves about the earth monthly

MENSES
The monthly discharge of blood, directly related to menstruation

MENSTRUATION
Refers to the monthly cycle, tied to the moon's cycles.

MONTH
a measure of time corresponding nearly to the period of the moon's revolution

The average length of a menstrual cycle is 28 days. However, a cycle can range in length from 21 days to about 30 days.

Your menstrual cycle is the time from the first day of your menstrual period until the first day of your next menstrual period. Every person's cycle is slightly different, but the process is the same.

Each month, as the moon goes through its phases, so does the female body as it prepares for its 28-30 day menstrual cycle.

MOON PHASES

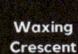 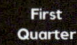 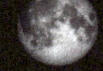   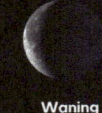 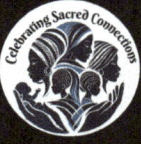

Waxing Crescent | First Quarter | Waxing Gibous | Full moon | Waning Gibous | Third Quarter | Waning Crescent

Vaginal Health
Womb Foods

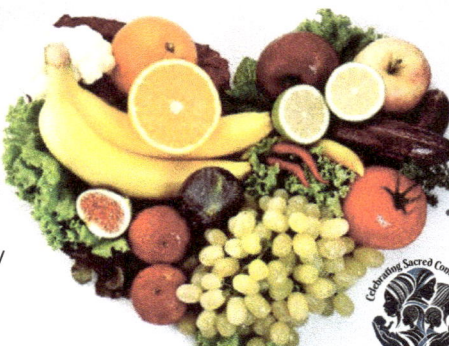

FRUITS:
- **Citrus fruits, guava, strawberries, kiwifruit, green and red peppers and broccoli** are rich in vitamin C which boosts immune system

VEGETABLES:
- **Avocado** contains B6 and potassium and support healthy vaginal walls; also helps with the libido.
- **Spinach, kale, cabbage, salad, Swiss chard, collards and other leafy greens** help with the circulation and prevent vaginal dryness.

Garlic has allicin, an active ingredient, that has antimicrobial and antifungal properties

PROBIOTICS:
- **Fermented foods like natural yogurt (or Greek yogurt), miso, kimchi, sauerkrauts and kefir** maintain vaginal pH at its slightly acidic level, and wards off yeast infections.

DRINKS:
- Water: hydrates the vaginal membrane
- Cranberries acidify urine and balance the pH of the vaginal area.

SEEDS & NUTS:
- **Sunflower seeds, almonds, walnuts, hazelnuts, & oils pumpkin seeds**, and oils derived from these nuts. Are rich in zinc. Essential mineral regulates the menstrual cycle.

All about my favorite womb care foods and how I am sure to include them in my diet:

WELCOME
TO WOMBMANHOOD

Becoming a wombman (woman) is an amazing experience and journey. This is an important time in your life, the beginning of many new experiences.

The life cycle and the monthly menstrual cycle are important aspects of living with the gift of womanhood.

This and other cycles are actually gifts from your Creator. Think of day and night, the seasons of the year, and birthdays --all cycles

The Creator of all systems of knowledge created you to be honored and celebrated and this beautiful cycle is one way to celebrate you.

Each of us is a scientist and our bodies are our labs. Let's study. Our labs will reveal much to us.

Celebrate and enjoy each stage of your development, knowing that each one is a gift and a blessing from The Creator.

THINK ABOUT HOW YOU HONOR YOUR SACRED WOMBMANHOOD.

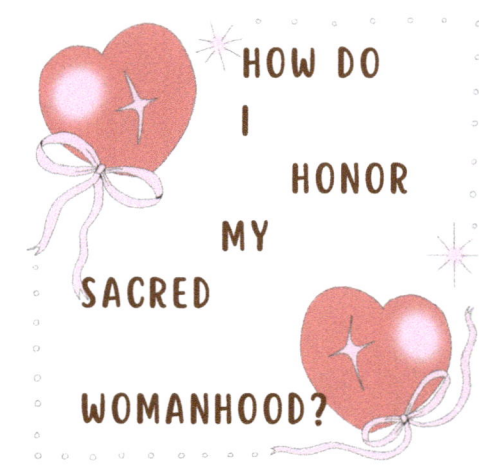

HOW DO I HONOR MY SACRED WOMANHOOD?

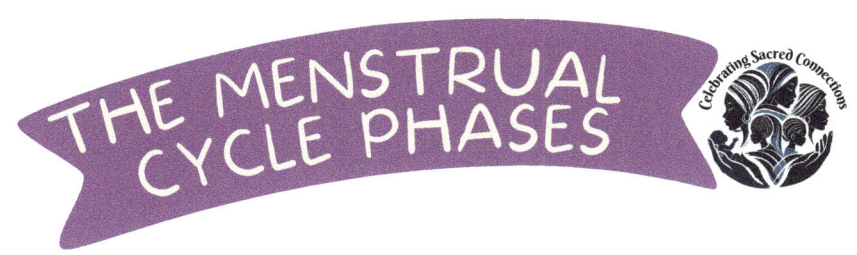
THE MENSTRUAL CYCLE PHASES

Each month, the lining of your uterus breaks down and sheds. This is menstruation. Menstruation is also known by the terms menses, menstrual period, menstrual cycle or period. The monthly shedding of the lining of your uterus appears as blood. Menstrual blood is partly blood and partly tissue from the inside of your uterus. The blood flows from your uterus through your cervix and out of your body through your vagina.

Luteal Phase: The luteal phase begins just after ovulation and ends when you start your period. If the egg is not fertilized, the endometrium (the layer of uterine tissue) begins to break down. The hormone levels decrease as the body prepares for a menstrual cycle.

The menses phase: The menses phase or bleeding days is the time when the lining of your uterus sheds through your vagina if pregnancy has not occurred.

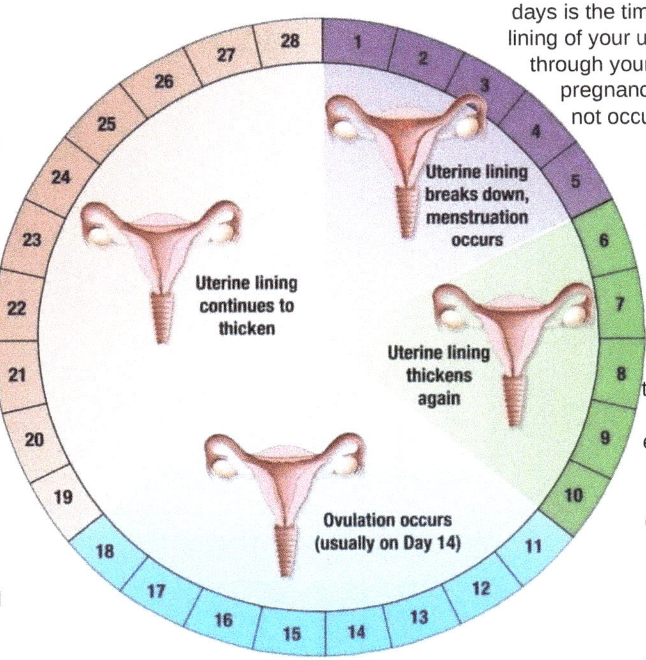

Follicular Phase. The follicular phase is when the level of the hormone estrogen rises, which causes the lining of your uterus (the endometrium) to grow and thicken. The ovaries produce around 5 to 20 small sacs called follicles.

Ovulatory Phase: The ovulatory phase begins when the ovary releases a mature egg. Your egg leaves your ovary and begins to travel through your fallopian tubes to your uterus. The egg travels down the fallopian tube toward the uterus to be fertilized. The level of the hormone progesterone rises to help prepare your uterine lining for pregnancy It lasts about 24 hours. After a day, the egg will die or dissolve if it is not fertilized. .

Menstrual Phase

"I release what no longer serves me, making space for renewal and growth."

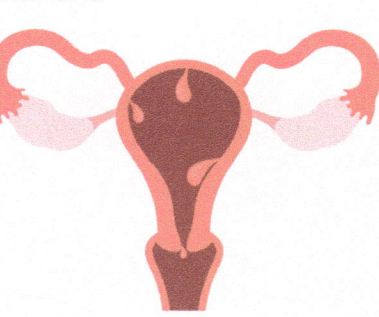

The menstrual phase is the start of your cycle when your body sheds the uterine lining. Hormones like estrogen and progesterone are at their lowest, which can lead to fatigue and discomfort.

Things to Do:
- **Rest:** Focus on restorative activities, like meditation or gentle yoga, to manage discomforts or low energy.
- **Self-Care:** Warm baths, heating pads, and plenty of sleep can help reduce discomfort.
- **Journaling:** This is a great time for self-reflection and setting intentions for the upcoming cycle.

What to Eat:
- **Iron-Rich Foods:** Due to blood loss, you need to replenish iron levels. Foods like leafy greens, lentils, red meat, and beans are excellent.
- **Hydrating Foods:** Water-rich fruits (like watermelon or cucumber) and herbal teas can help alleviate bloating and discomfort.
- **Anti-Inflammatory Foods:** Ginger, turmeric, and omega-3 fatty acids (found in fish and flaxseeds) can help reduce cramps.

Honor the Menstrual Phase by answering the questions and writing each day.

Today I write about how I am feeling physically and emotionally. What do I need to nurture myself during this time?

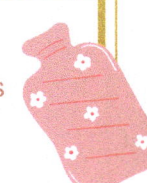

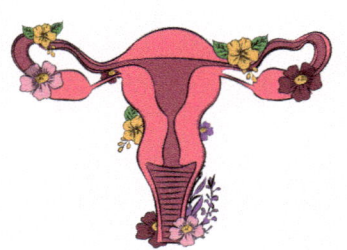

How do I describe my feelings? How do I connect with my intuition and honor it?

Here is how I can honor my need for rest and renewal during this phase.

What are ways that I demonstrate that I regard my womb as precious?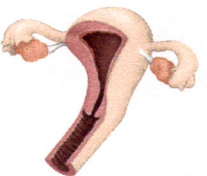

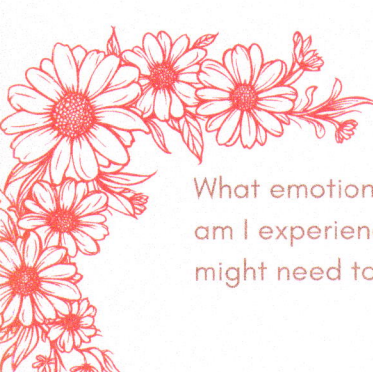
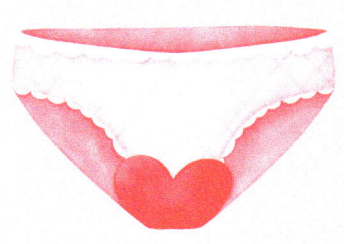

What emotions or thoughts am I experiencing that I might need to let go of?

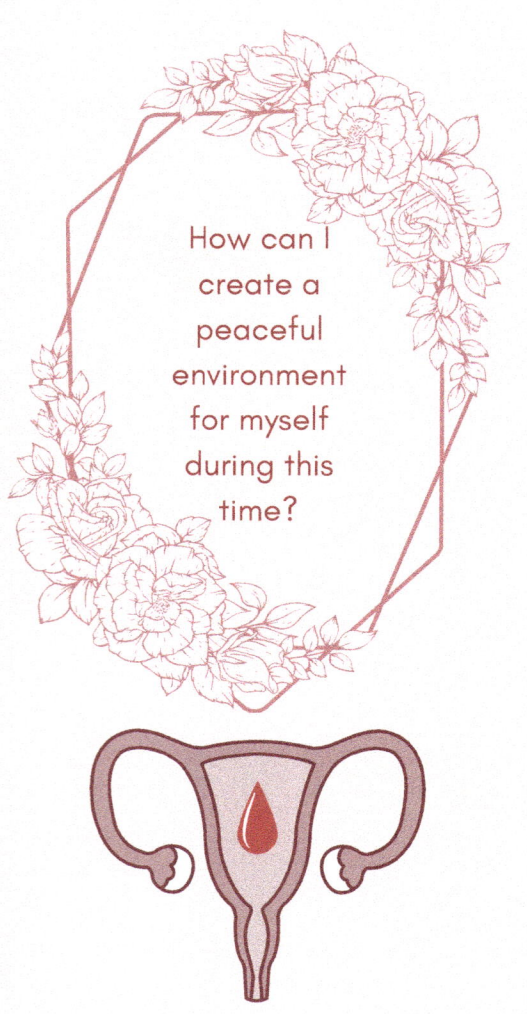

How can I create a peaceful environment for myself during this time?

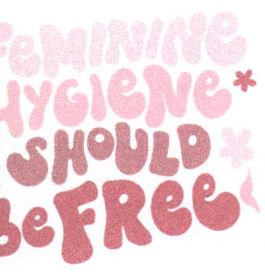

Am I conscious of the natural products I use during my bleed days? Why is it important to use products that benefit my body and my wellness?

How am I responding to the thoughts or feelings about menstruation that come up for me during this time?

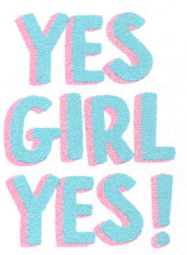

How do I take time to be still, observe and track the cycle, checking for color, clots, texture, (thick or thin), odor, changes day to day, period to period?

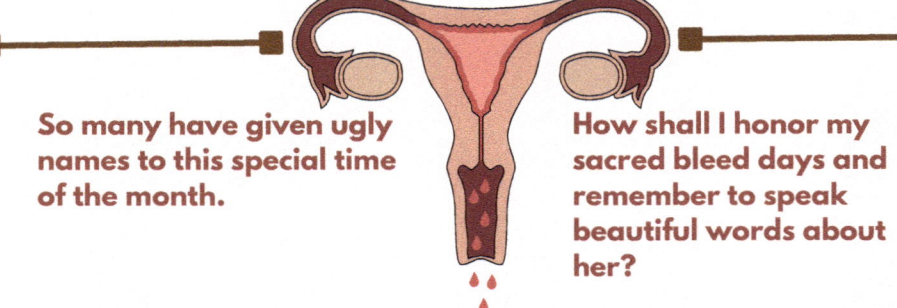

So many have given ugly names to this special time of the month.

How shall I honor my sacred bleed days and remember to speak beautiful words about her?

Follicular Phase

"I am confident, full of vitality, and ready to take on the world."

After menstruation, estrogen levels rise, and the body begins to prepare for ovulation. This is typically the phase where energy starts increasing.

THINGS TO DO:
- **Exercise:** You may feel energized, so it's a great time to engage in more intense physical activities like cardio, strength training, or even trying something new like dance or cycling.
- **Set Goals**: Your mental clarity and motivation might be heightened, making this a great time to plan or start new projects.
- **Socialize:** If you feel more outgoing, it's a good time for social events or networking.

WHAT TO EAT:
- **Protein and Fiber-Rich Foods:** Support energy and blood sugar stability with foods like quinoa, eggs, legumes, and seeds.
- **Cruciferous Vegetables:** Broccoli, cauliflower, and kale support healthy estrogen metabolism.
- **Fermented Foods:** Sauerkraut, kimchi, and yogurt help maintain gut health and support digestion during hormonal changes.

Pay attention to your body, thoughts, and heart during the Follicular Phase and answer the questions and write each day.

What new ideas or projects am I excited to explore during this phase?

How can I harness the energy and motivation I feel to move toward my goals?

What intentions do I want to set for the upcoming weeks?

What new ideas or projects am I excited to explore during this phase?

How can I channel my creativity into something meaningful or fulfilling?

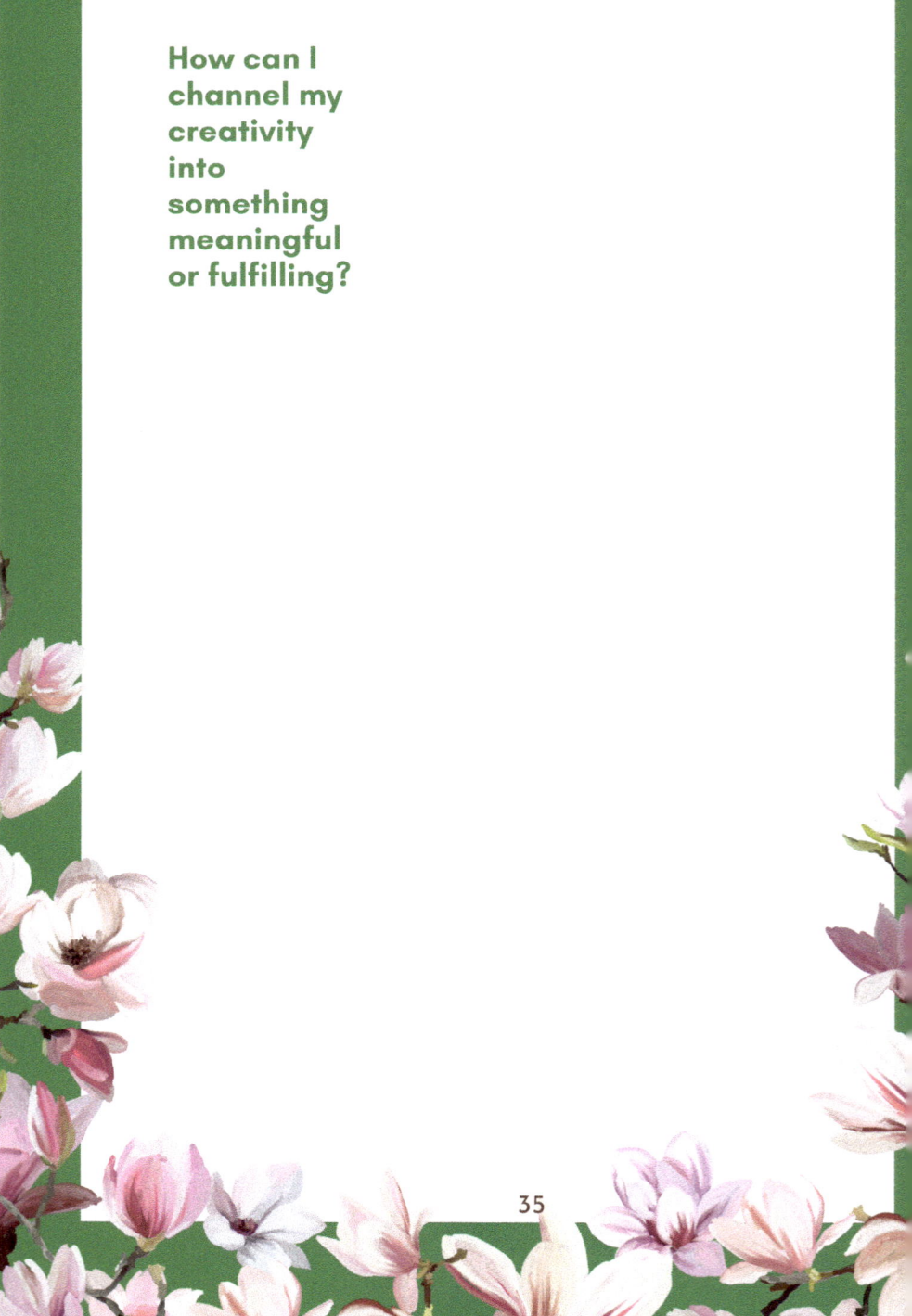

What steps can I take to build momentum in areas of my life that feel stagnant?

How do I want to approach challenges or opportunities with a fresh perspective?

What inspires me right now, and how can I cultivate that inspiration further?

What self-care practices can I incorporate to support my rising energy levels?

How can I channel my renewed energy into areas of my life that need growth or attention?

"The power to manifest lies within me, and I am in alignment with my highest self."

Ovulatory Phase

Ovulatory Phase is when the mature egg is released from the ovary. Estrogen peaks and testosterone rises slightly, leading to increased energy, libido, and confidence.

THINGS TO DO:
- **Be Active:** Engage in high-energy activities like running, hiking, or dancing.
- **Social Activities:** This is a great time for social gatherings, important meetings, or public speaking, as communication skills may be heightened.
- **Creative Pursuits:** Harness the burst of energy for creative projects or brainstorming sessions.

WHAT TO EAT:
- **Antioxidant-Rich Foods:** Support egg health with foods like berries, spinach, and dark chocolate.
- **Zinc and Magnesium:** Help regulate hormonal balance with pumpkin seeds, chickpeas, and almonds.
- **Vitamin C:** Boost immunity and overall health with citrus fruits, bell peppers, and strawberries

Honor the Ovulatory Phase by answering the questions and writing each day.

What do I feel most confident and empowered about right now?

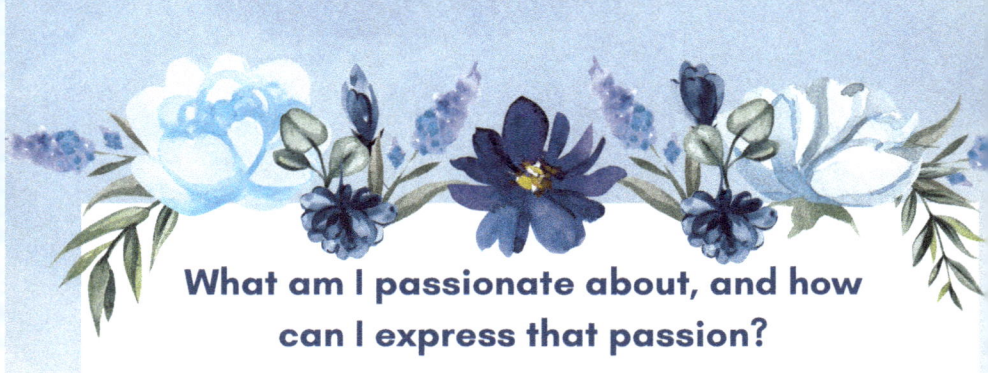

What am I passionate about, and how can I express that passion?

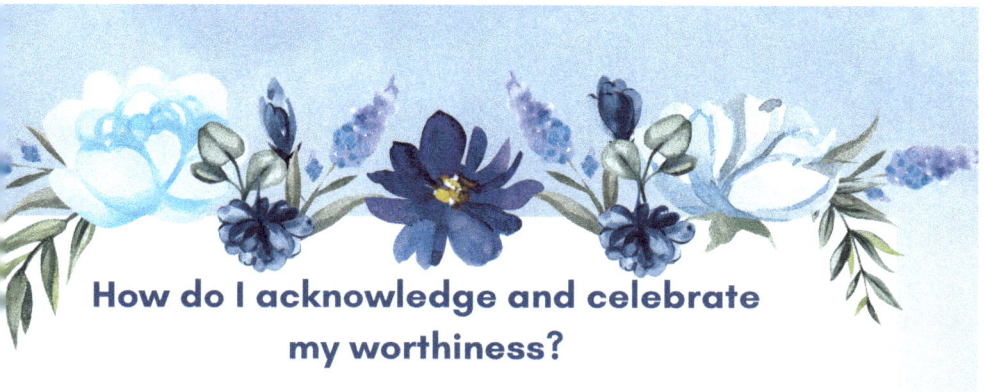

How do I acknowledge and celebrate my worthiness?

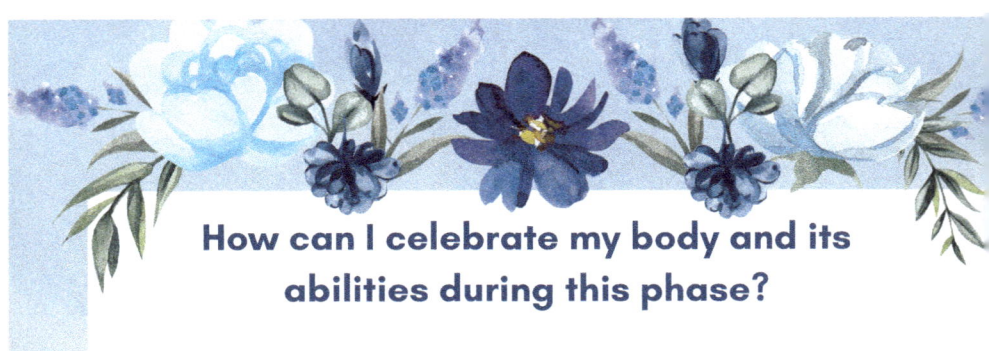

How can I celebrate my body and its abilities during this phase?

How can I use this high-energy phase to pursue creative projects, work goals, or social connections? What ideas are bubbling up that excite me?

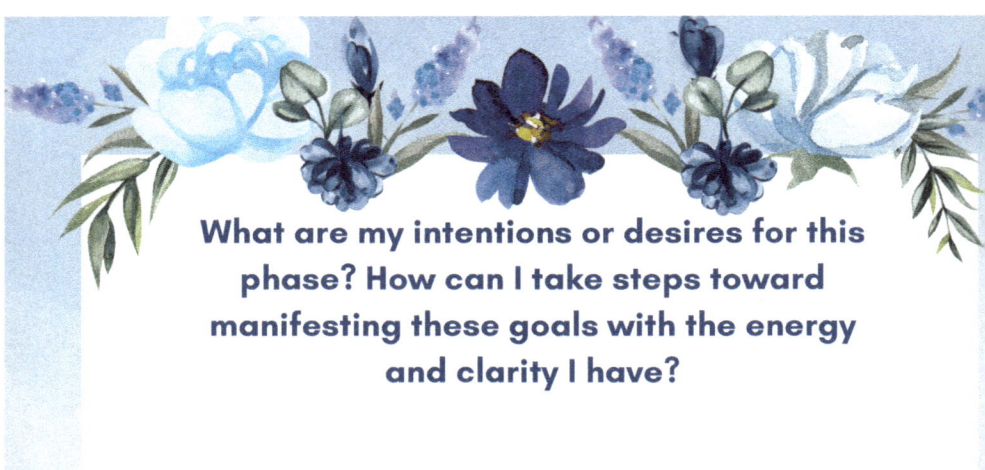

What are my intentions or desires for this phase? How can I take steps toward manifesting these goals with the energy and clarity I have?

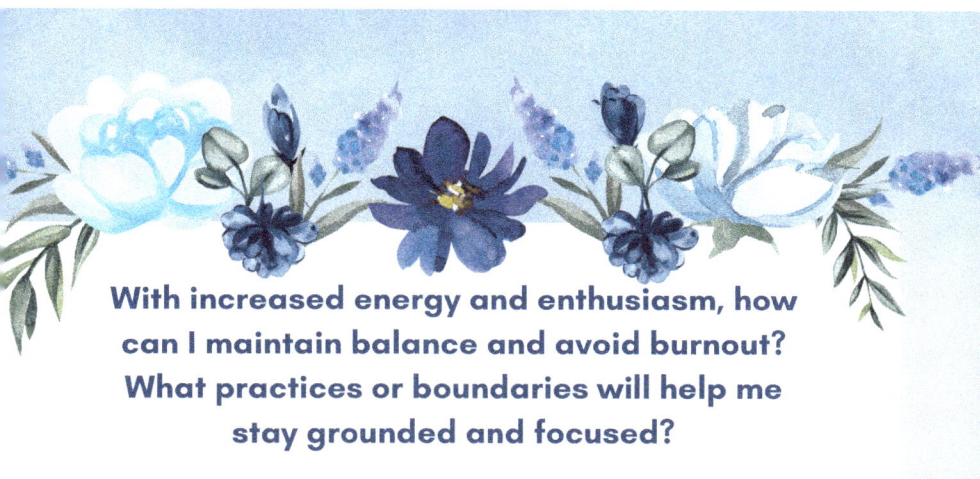

With increased energy and enthusiasm, how can I maintain balance and avoid burnout? What practices or boundaries will help me stay grounded and focused?

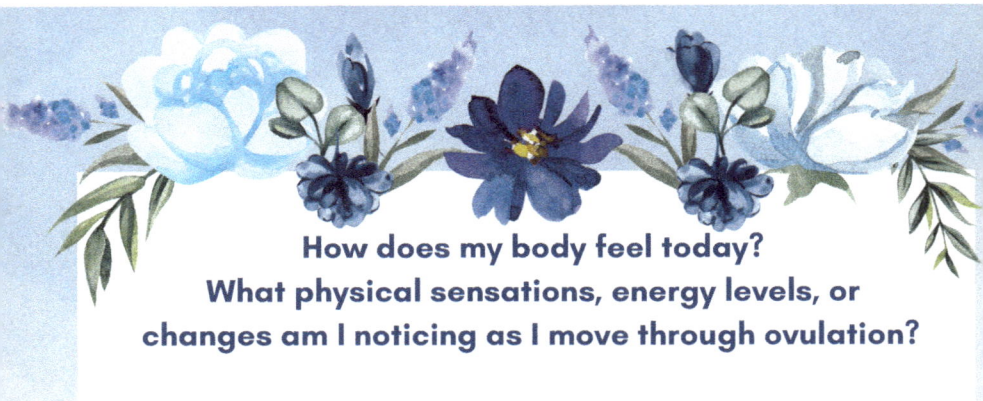

**How does my body feel today?
What physical sensations, energy levels, or changes am I noticing as I move through ovulation?**

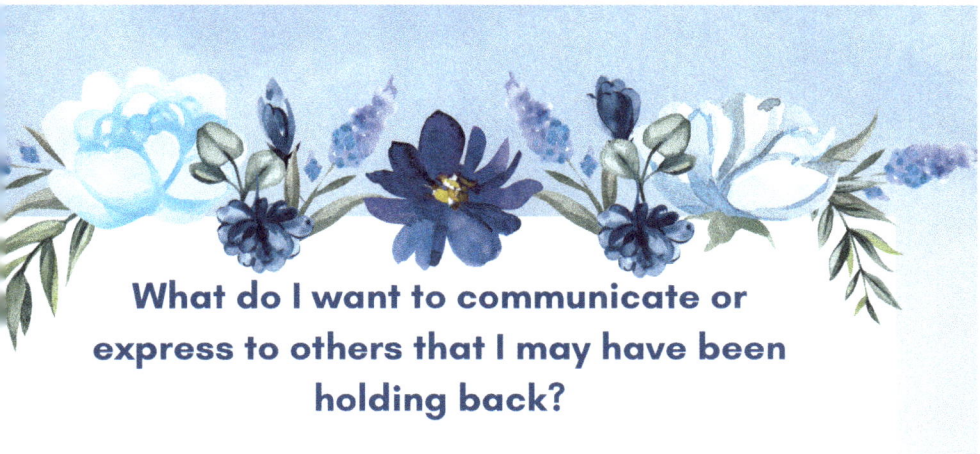

What do I want to communicate or express to others that I may have been holding back?

Luteal Phase

After ovulation, progesterone levels rise to prepare for potential pregnancy. If the egg is not fertilized, hormone levels drop.

"In a world of constant change, I trust the cycles of my body to lead me to peace and balance."

THINGS TO DO:
- **Low-Intensity Exercise:** Switch to more gentle exercises like yoga, walking, or Pilates if you feel sluggish.
- **Relax and Reflect:** Practice stress-relief techniques like deep breathing, meditation, or journaling to manage mood changes.
- **Tackle Small Tasks:** Energy might dip, so focus on smaller tasks and self-care routines.

WHAT TO EAT:
- **Complex Carbs:** Support mood and energy with whole grains, sweet potatoes, and legumes.
- **Magnesium-Rich Foods:** Reduce bloating and soothe muscles with spinach, bananas, and nuts.
- **Healthy Fats:** Support hormone production with avocados, chia seeds, and oily fish like salmon.
- **Herbal Teas:** Chamomile or peppermint tea can soothe digestive issues and reduce bloating.

Write your heart out as you answer the questions each day during this phase.

How can I create a balance between productivity and rest as my energy shifts?

What tasks or projects can I complete to bring a sense of closure before the next cycle begins?

What challenges or emotions have come up for me recently, and how can I process them with compassion?

What small rituals or routines help me stay grounded and centered during this time?

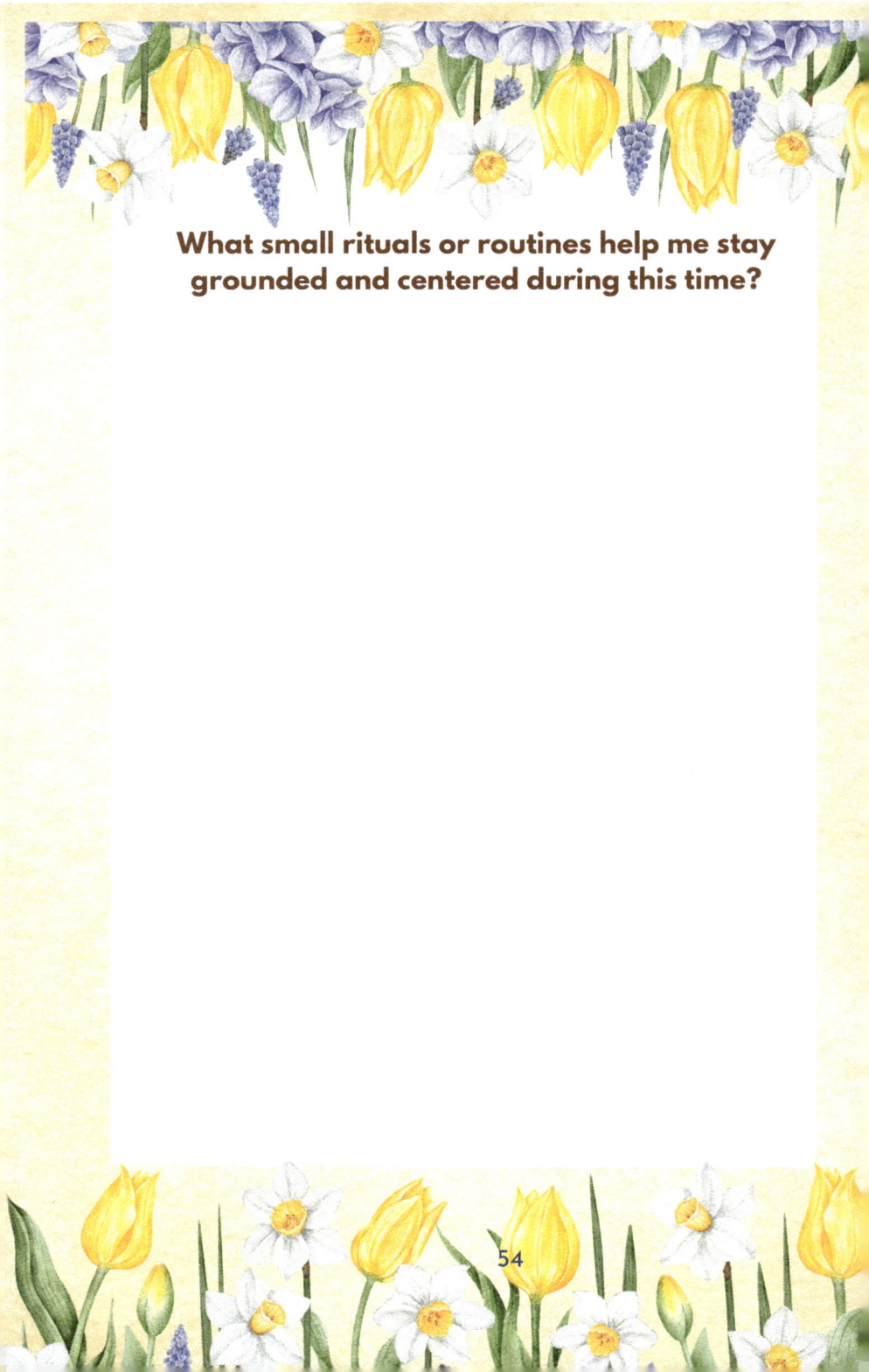

How can I practice self-care to manage any physical or emotional discomfort I may feel?

What boundaries do I need to set to protect my well-being during this phase?

What emotions or thoughts are surfacing, and how can I process them constructively?

How can I practice self-care to manage any physical or emotional discomfort I may feel?

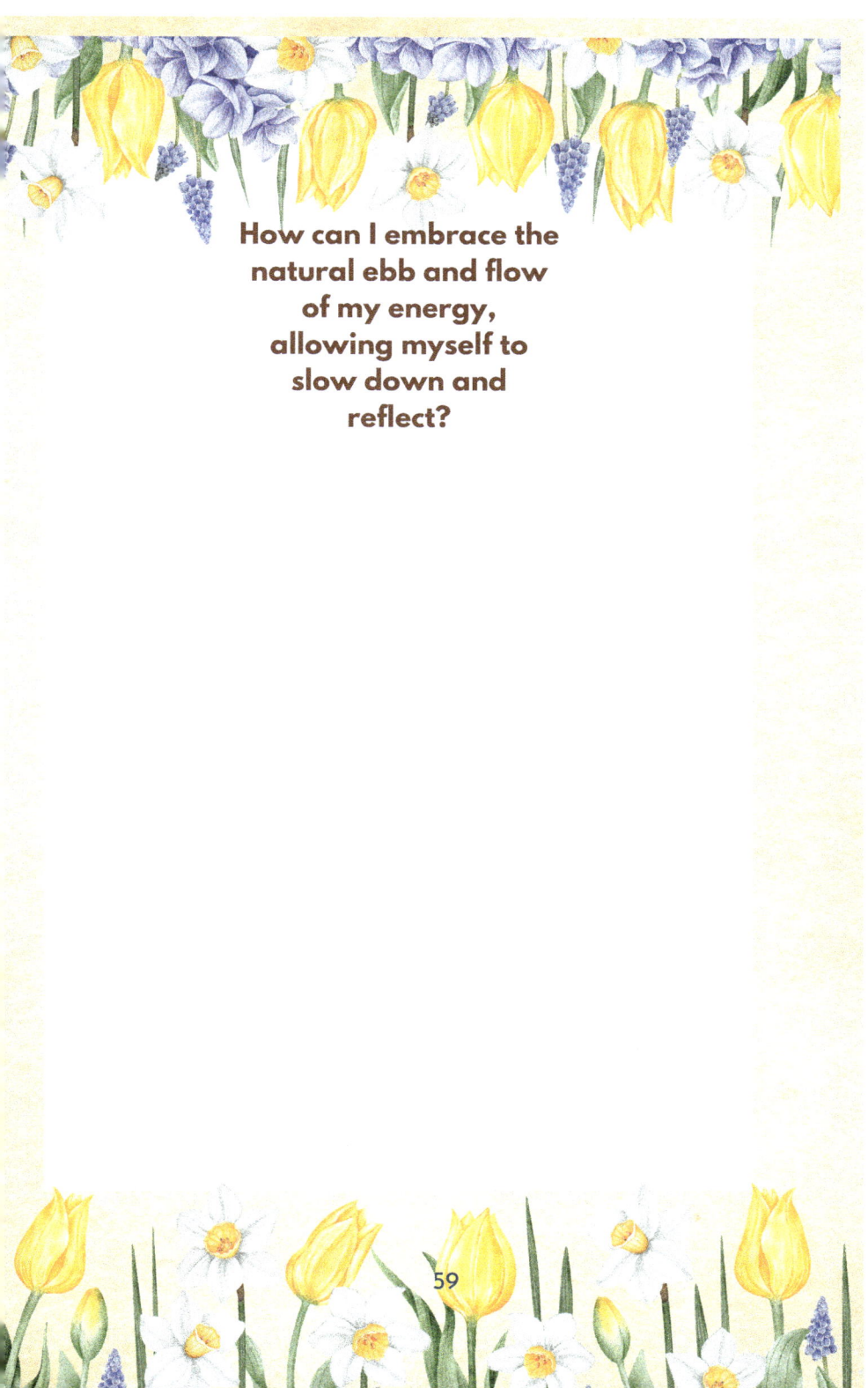

How can I embrace the natural ebb and flow of my energy, allowing myself to slow down and reflect?

What do I need to let go of to enter the next phase with clarity and focus?

WRITING prompts

During the selected phase, try writing using one of the prompts.

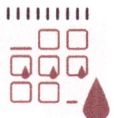
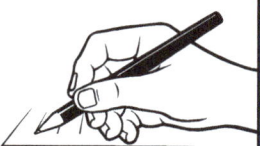

MENSTRUAL
What does my body need most right now, and how can I provide it?

MENSTRUAL
How can I honor my need for rest and renewal during this phase?

MENSTRUAL
Design a robot that helps make breakfast for your family each day.

FOLLICULAR
What goals or desires am I ready to manifest, and what steps can I take to achieve them?

FOLLICULAR
What are my G-d given gifts that I can develop and nurture my feminine attributes\ energies\ principles?

FOLLICULAR
What am I passionate about, and how can I express that passion?

OVULATORY
What makes me feel vibrant and alive, and how can I incorporate more of that into my life?

OVULATORY
How can I embrace my natural inclinations and take action on what matters most to me?

OVULATORY
How can I practice gratitude for the abundance and opportunities in my life?

LUTEAL
What small rituals or routines help me stay grounded and centered during this time?

LUTEAL
How can I practice self-care to manage any physical or emotional discomfort I may feel?

LUTEAL
How can I practice mindfulness and stay present with my emotions?

Self-Care Rules

We are all gifted with inner wisdom, and it is important to share our gifts.

Spending time with other women in safe and supported environments is incredible and rejuvenating. It regulates the inner self.

Being in nature is essential to getting grounded and connected with the elements, thus enabling access to deep intuitive wisdom, boundless energy and endless inspiration

Health is dependent on balance. Work with subtle energies of the body and mind to create a better functioning organism.

We have lost our self-reliance when it comes to health care and, thus, we have forgotten how to properly take care of ourselves .

PERIOD PARTY PLANNING

Planning a period party is a unique and empowering way to celebrate menstruation and raise awareness. Celebrating a person's period (whether it is the first one or years of having a period) can be a positive and empowering experience. A period party can help remove the stigma surrounding menstruation and create an environment of support and education. We pray that you find great benefit in our step-by-step guide to help you plan a period party

THE EVENT

Event Date and Time:
- Preferred date(s) and time for the party?

Guest List:
- How many people are you planning to invite?
- Are the guests all of a certain age group or mixed ages?

Theme and Purpose:
- Is there a specific theme for the party?
- What is the main purpose of the event (e.g., celebration, education, support)?

Discussion Topics:
- What key topics do you want to cover (menstrual health, hygiene, myths)?
- Will there be a Q&A session or open discussion?

Venue and Decorations
- Venue:
  - Where will the party be held (home, community center, outdoor space)?
  - Do you need to book the venue in advance?
- Decorations:
  - What type of decorations are you considering (banners, balloons, flowers)?
  - Are there any specific colors or symbols you want to use?

ACTIVITIES AND ENTERTAINMENT

Activities:
- How will you honor elders, significant men- father figures, uncles, spiritual leaders, etc
- What activities do you want to include (games, crafts, educational sessions)?
- Will there be any guest speakers or demonstrations?

Entertainment:
- Are you planning any entertainment (music, dance, performances)?
- Do you need to hire any entertainers or musicians?

Food and Drinks
- What type of womb foods and drinks will be served (snacks, meals, tea (hot or cold), etc.)?
- Are there any dietary restrictions or preferences to consider?

Special Menstrual-Themed Treats:
- Will you have any special treats or themed food items?

Informational Material:
- Are you providing any educational materials (pamphlets, books, videos)?
- Do you need to prepare or source these materials in advance?

Party Favors and Gifts
- Are you planning to give out any party favors or gifts?
- What type of favors (menstrual product samples, self-care items)?
- Will there be any keepsakes or mementos for guests to take home?

BUDGET & RESOURCES

Budget:
- What is your overall budget for the party?
- How will the budget be allocated (venue, food, decorations, entertainment)?

Sponsors and Donations:
- Are you seeking any sponsorships or donations?
- Who will you approach for potential contributions?

Logistics and Coordination
Invitations:
- How will you send out invitations (digital, paper)?
- When do you plan to send them out?

RSVP and Follow-Up:
- How will you manage RSVPs?
- Will you send reminders or follow-ups to guests?

Event Day Coordination:
- Who will help you set up and manage the event on the day?
- Do you need any volunteers or additional staff?

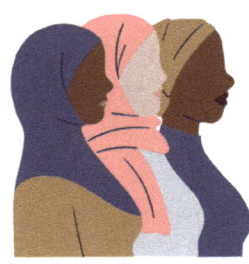

Spending time with other women in safe and supported environment is incredible and rejuvenating. It regulates the inner self.

Who are the sisters in my sacred sisterhood and why?

Watch the moon. What do I see? What phase is it in, and how does it make me feel? What thoughts or emotions arise as I reflect on the moon's cycles and its connection to my own inner rhythms?

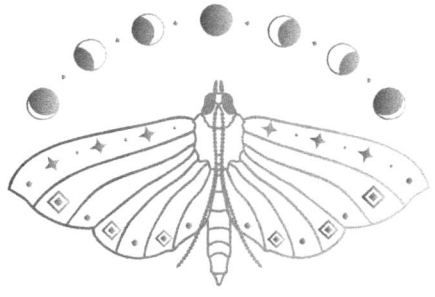

How can I align my energy with the moon's current phase—
whether it's a time for growth, release, or renewal?

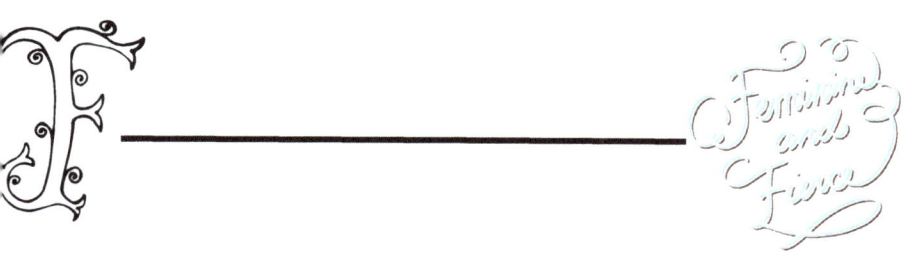

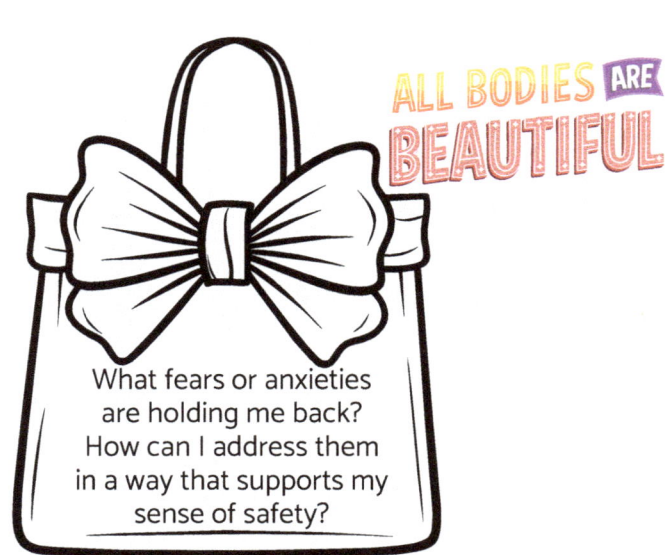

What fears or anxieties are holding me back? How can I address them in a way that supports my sense of safety?

ALL BODIES ARE BEAUTIFUL

What activities bring me joy and allow me to express my creativity? How can I make more time for them in my life?

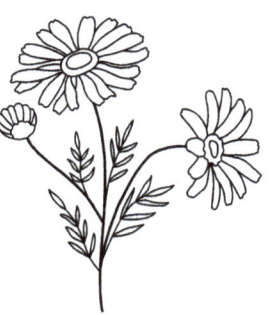

How do I express myself and communicate my thoughts and feelings? What can I do to communicate more effectively?

What truths am I hesitant to speak?
How can I find the courage to express them?

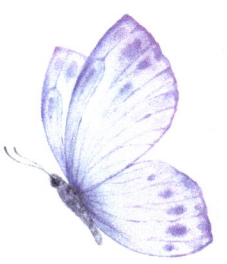

 How do I listen to others? What can I do to become a better listener and more attuned to others' needs?

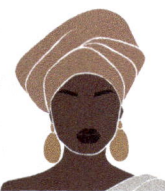 What do I learn about my body each time I go through the menstrual phases?

Which chakra feels most balanced and open right now? How does that manifest in my life?

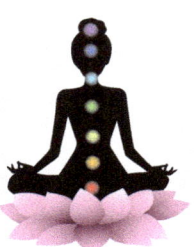

Which chakra feels blocked or out of balance? What practices can I use to heal and balance it?

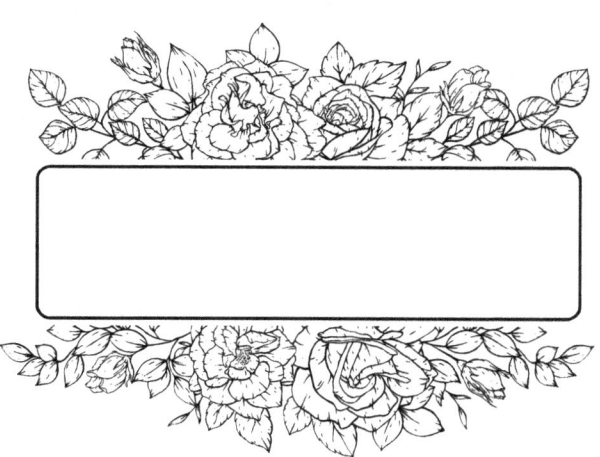

PERIOD TRACKER

NAME

	J	F	M	A	M	J	J	A	S	O	N	D
1												
2												
3												
4												
5												
6												
7												
8												
9												
10												
11												
12												
13												
14												
15												
16												
17												
18												
19												
20												
21												
22												
23												
24												
25												
26												
27												
28												
29												
30												
31												

SYMPTOMS KEY

- [ ] Spotting
- [ ] Light
- [ ] Medium
- [ ] Heavy
- [ ] Acne
- [ ] Cramps
- [ ] Cravings
- [ ] Fatigue
- [ ] Headache

THINGS TO AVOID

- [ ]
- [ ]
- [ ]
- [ ]
- [ ]

NOTES

_____
_____
_____
_____
_____
_____
_____

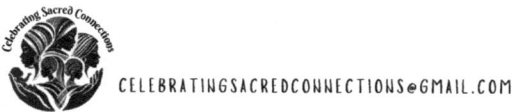

CELEBRATINGSACREDCONNECTIONS@GMAIL.COM

PERIOD TRACKER

NAME _____

	J	F	M	A	M	J	J	A	S	O	N	D
1												
2												
3												
4												
5												
6												
7												
8												
9												
10												
11												
12												
13												
14												
15												
16												
17												
18												
19												
20												
21												
22												
23												
24												
25												
26												
27												
28												
29												
30												
31												

SYMPTOMS KEY

- [ ] Spotting
- [ ] Light
- [ ] Medium
- [ ] Heavy
- [ ] Acne
- [ ] Cramps
- [ ] Cravings
- [ ] Fatigue
- [ ] Headache

THINGS TO AVOID

- [ ]
- [ ]
- [ ]
- [ ]
- [ ]

NOTES

_____
_____
_____
_____
_____
_____

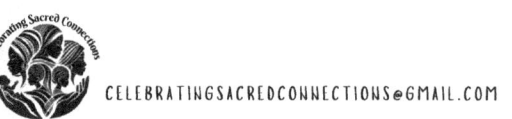

CELEBRATINGSACREDCONNECTIONS@GMAIL.COM

Month of: _____

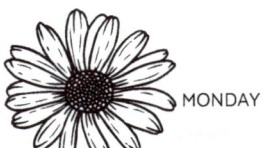 # MONTHLY PLANNER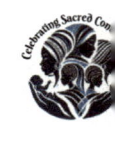

MONDAY　　TUESDAY　　WEDNESDAY　　THURSDAY　　FRIDAY　　SATURDAY

Mark the month and the days of the month on the calendar. For each day, keep track of your habits by answering the questions listed.

What I ate?

What I felt?

Chart the color of the blood during your cycle for each day of the cycle.

N⊙TES:

Month of: _____

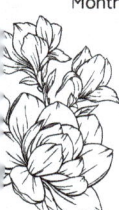

MONTHLY PLANNER

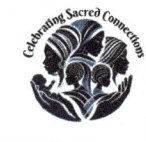

MONDAY   TUESDAY   WEDNESDAY   THURSDAY   FRIDAY   SATURDAY

Mark the month and the days of the month on the calendar. For each day, keep track of your habits by answering the questions listed.

What I ate?

What I felt?

Chart the color of the blood during your cycle for each bleed day of the cycle.

N·OTES:

MONTH OF: _____

MONTHLY PLANNER

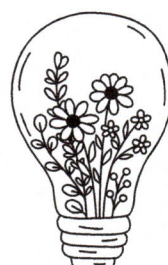

MONDAY   TUESDAY   WEDNESDAY   THURSDAY   FRIDAY   SATURDAY

Mark the month and the days of the month on the calendar. For each day, keep track of your habits by answering the questions listed.

What I ate?

What I felt?

Chart the color of the blood during your cycle for each day of the cycle.

NOTES:

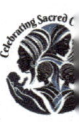

MONTH OF: _____

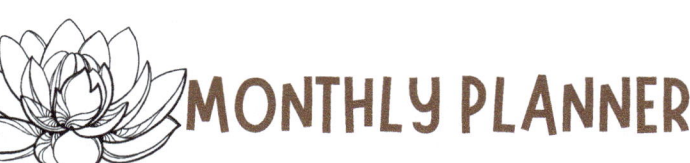
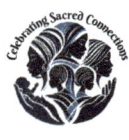

MONDAY	TUESDAY	WEDNESDAY	THURSDAY	FRIDAY	SATURDAY

NOTES:

Mark the month and the days of the month on the calendar. For each day, keep track of your habits by answering the questions listed.

What I ate?

What I felt?

Chart the color of the blood during your cycle for each day of the cycle.

NOTES:

MONTH OF: _____

MONTHLY PLANNER

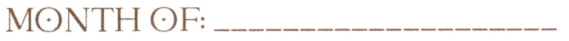

MONDAY	TUESDAY	WEDNESDAY	THURSDAY	FRIDAY	SATURDAY

NOTES:

Mark the month and the days of the month on the calendar. For each day, keep track of your habits by answering the questions listed.

What I ate?

What I felt?

Chart the color of the blood during your cycle for each day of the cycle.

NOTES:

MONTH OF: _____

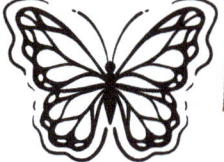

MONTHLY PLANNER

| MONDAY | TUESDAY | WEDNESDAY | THURSDAY | FRIDAY | SATURDAY |

NOTES:

Mark the month and the days of the month on the calendar. For each day, keep track of your habits by answering the questions listed.

What I ate?

What I felt?

Chart the color of the blood during your cycle for each day of the cycle.

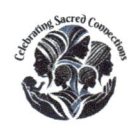

MONTH OF: _____

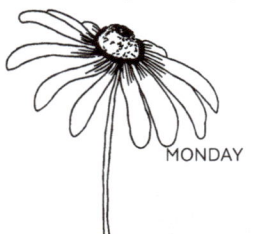

MONTHLY PLANNER

MONDAY	TUESDAY	WEDNESDAY	THURSDAY	FRIDAY	SATURDAY

NOTES:

Mark the month and the days of the month on the calendar. For each day, keep track of your habits by answering the questions listed.

What I ate?

What I felt?

Chart the color of the blood during your cycle for each day of the cycle.

NOTES:

MONTH OF: _____

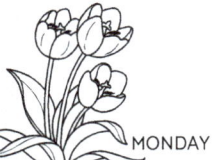

MONTHLY PLANNER

| MONDAY | TUESDAY | WEDNESDAY | THURSDAY | FRIDAY | SATURDAY |

NOTES:

Mark the month and the days of the month on the calendar. For each day, keep track of your habits by answering the questions listed.

What I ate?

What I felt?

Chart the color of the blood during your cycle for each day of the cycle.

NOTES:

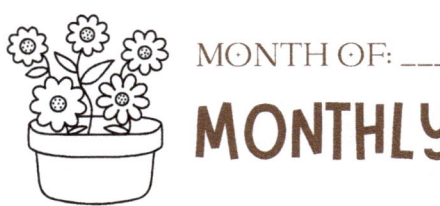

MONTH OF: _____

MONTHLY PLANNER

| MONDAY | TUESDAY | WEDNESDAY | THURSDAY | FRIDAY | SATURDAY |

NOTES:

Mark the month and the days of the month on the calendar. For each day, keep track of your habits by answering the questions listed.

What I ate?

What I felt?

Chart the color of the blood during your cycle for each day of the cycle.

NOTES:

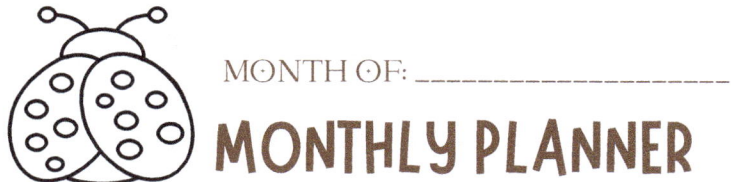

MONTH OF: _____

MONTHLY PLANNER

MONDAY	TUESDAY	WEDNESDAY	THURSDAY	FRIDAY	SATURDAY

NOTES:

Mark the month and the days of the month on the calendar. For each day, keep track of your habits by answering the questions listed.

What I ate?

What I felt?

Chart the color of the blood during your cycle for each day of the cycle.

NOTES:

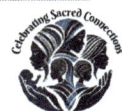

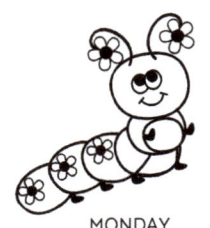

MONTH OF: _____

MONTHLY PLANNER

MONDAY	TUESDAY	WEDNESDAY	THURSDAY	FRIDAY	SATURDAY

NOTES:

Mark the month and the days of the month on the calendar. For each day, keep track of your habits by answering the questions listed.

What I ate?

What I felt?

Chart the color of the blood during your cycle for each day of the cycle.

NOTES:

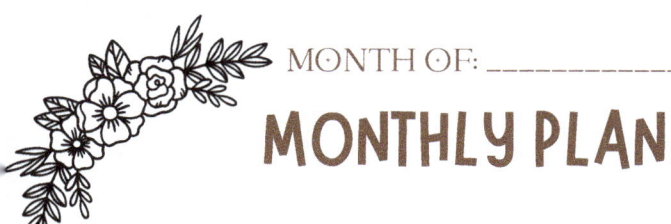

MONTH OF: _____

MONTHLY PLANNER

MONDAY	TUESDAY	WEDNESDAY	THURSDAY	FRIDAY	SATURDAY

NOTES:

Mark the month and the days of the month on the calendar. For each day, keep track of your habits by answering the questions listed.

What I ate?

What I felt?

Chart the color of the blood during your cycle for each day of the cycle.

NOTES:

MONTH OF: _____

MONTHLY PLANNER

MONDAY	TUESDAY	WEDNESDAY	THURSDAY	FRIDAY	SATURDAY

NOTES:

Mark the month and the days of the month on the calendar. For each day, keep track of your habits by answering the questions listed.

What I ate?

What I felt?

Chart the color of the blood during your cycle for each day of the cycle.

NOTES:

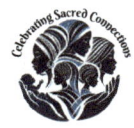

SET AN ACTION! PLAN

An action plan is like a step-by-step guide that helps you reach a goal. Think of it like a map for a fun adventure! Now that you've completed your Sacred Menstrual Cycle Journal, it's time to make an action plan!

This is where you think about how to take care of yourself during each part of your cycle. Look back at your journal and write down the things that made you feel strong, calm, and happy. Then, decide what you'll do in the months and years ahead to make sure you're rested, eating well, and having fun.

You can set small goals like getting extra sleep during your period or doing something creative when you feel energized. Your action plan is like a guide to help you feel your best through each phase!

Joyful

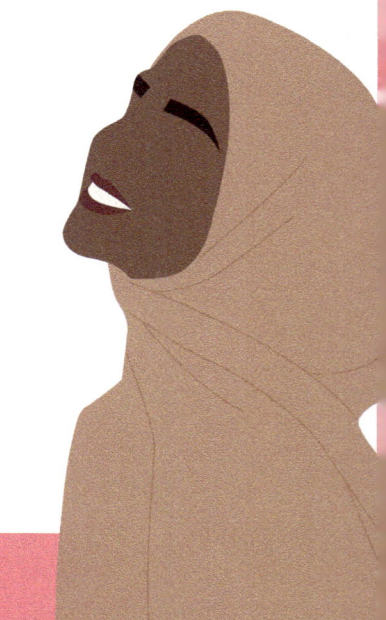

Empowered

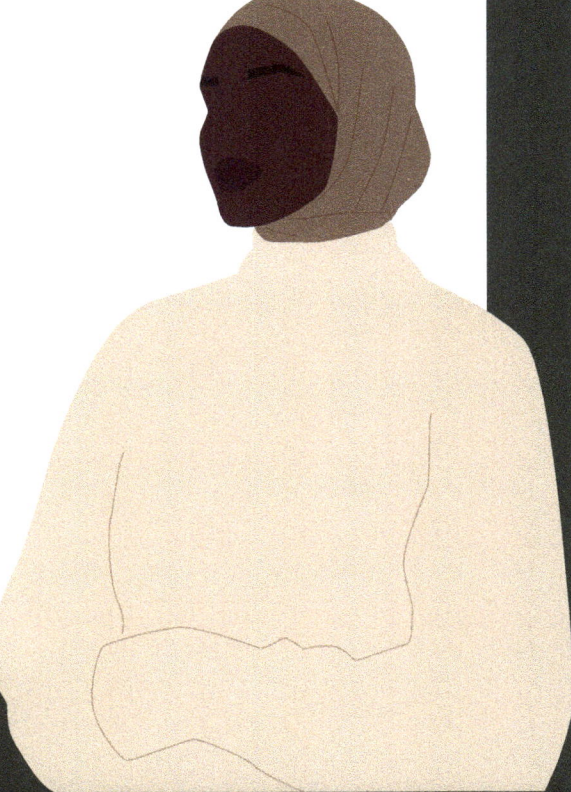

Brave

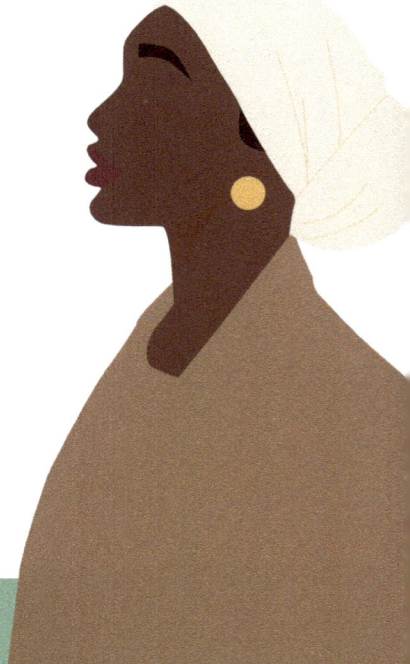

The male and female are similar with vast degrees of differences. What are the immediate similarities you notice? What are the differences?

THE MALE Reproductive System

SEMINAL VESICLE
produces seminal fluid that makes up majority of the semen

VAS DEFERENS
a tube that transports mature sperm out of the testes

PROSTATE GLAND
also poduces fluid for transporting sperm

TESTIS
produces sperm and testosterone

PENIS
external male reproductive organ

URETHRA
a tube from the bladder to the penis, where urine and sperm passes

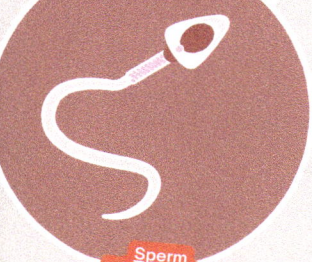

Sperm — male sex cell

THE FEMALE Reproductive System

FALLOPIAN TUBE — where the sperm and egg cell often meet during fertilization; connects the ovary to the uterus

UTERUS — prepares its lining to nourish a fertilized ovum until birth; if there is no fertilization, the lining sheds during mentstuation

CERVIX — passage to and from the uterus

OVARY — produces and stores egg cells

VAGINA — a muscular opening where menstrual blood leaves or a baby goes out during birth

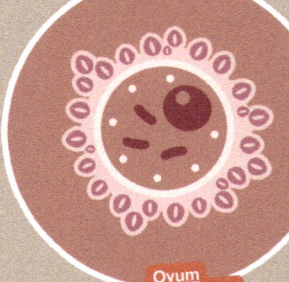

Ovum — female sex cell

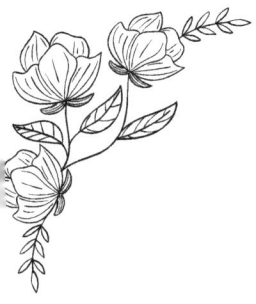
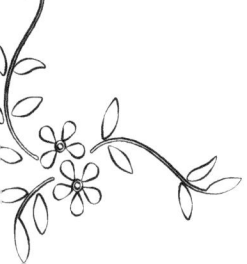
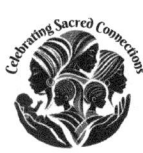

celebratingsacredconnections@gmail.com

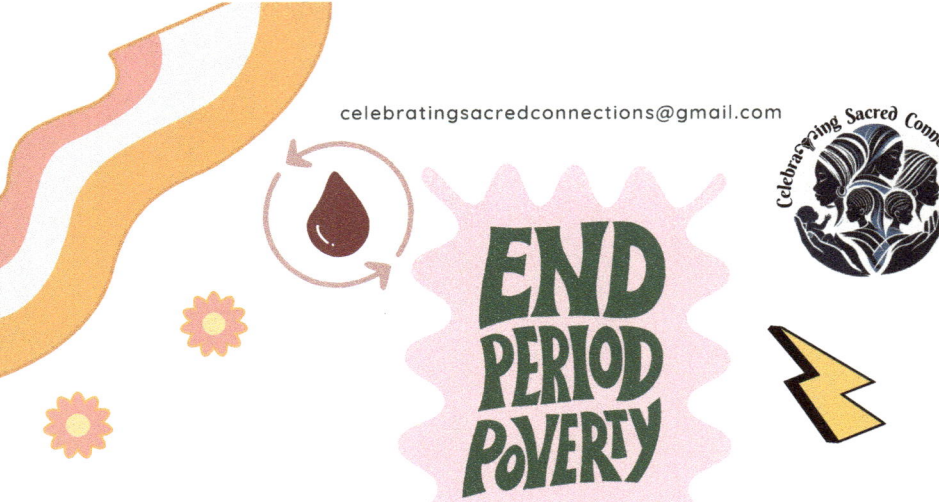

celebratingsacredconnections@gmail.com

about the authors

Celebrating Sacred Connections empowers women by celebrating feminine strength, health, and hygiene from ages 4 to 104. Founded by retired nurse Adilah Muhammad and education consultant Qur'an Shakir, both with 30+ years of experience, the organization offers wombmen-centered celebrations, retreats, and coaching. Specializing in yoni health, postpartum healing, and rites of passage programs, they provide tailored events like coming-of-age parties, yoni steaming sessions, bridal pampering, and wombmen's circles. Their mission is to honor the divine feminine and inspire love for the Yoni and true G'd-given femininity.

celebratingsacredconnections@gmail.com
www.celebratingsacredconnections.org

www.ingramcontent.com/pod-product-compliance
Lightning Source LLC
Chambersburg PA
CBHW052037030426
42337CB00027B/5045